Breastfeeding Facts
for Fathers

Platypus Media

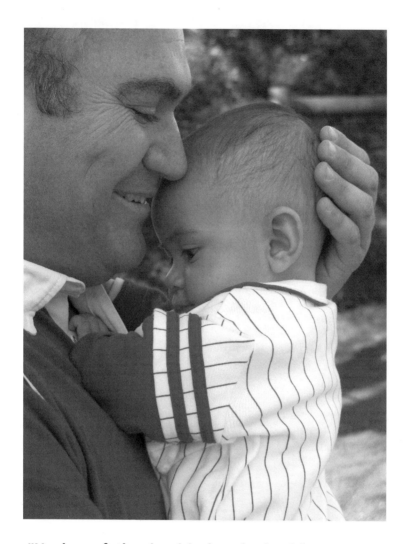

"Having a father is critical to the healthy
development of a child.
Being a father is critical to the healthy
development of a man."

Terrence Real, *How Can I Get Through to You:
Reconnecting Men and Women*

This booklet is not intended to be a replacement for advice from your health care provider. Readers and their families should consult a professional health care provider on a regular basis. This book is not meant to be a substitute for your doctor. It is a general informational guide and reference source. No medical or legal responsibility is assumed by the author or publisher.

Executive Editor: Dia L. Michels
Senior Editor: Jessica Wilde
Project Design: Deb Stover, Image Media, Sterling, VA

Copyright © 2009 Platypus Media, LLC

Gift Paperback Edition • June 2009
  English– ISBN: 978-1-930775-49-7
  Spanish–ISBN: 978-1-930775-42 8

Also available in other formats:
  eBook Edition • June 2009
  English–ISBN: 978-1-930775-50-3
  Second Edition Booklet* • June 2009
  English– ISBN: 978-1-930775-12-1
  Spanish– ISBN: 978-1-930775-42-8
    [Originally published in 2003 as ISBN: 978-1-930775-17-2]
    *Same content as Gift Paperback Book in a lighter, thinner version

  Abridged Edition** • June 2009
  English– ISBN: 978-1-930775-51-0
  Spanish–ISBN: 978-1-930775-54-1
    ** Shortened version (16 pages), easier reading level

Mixed Sources
Product group from well-managed forests and other controlled sources
www.fsc.org   Cert no. SW-COC-002283
© 1996 Forest Stewardship Council
FSC

Distributed to the book trade in the United States by:
  National Book Network
  (301) 459-3366 / Toll free: 800-787-6859 / Fax: 301-429-5746
  CustServ@nbnbooks.com / www.nbnbooks.com

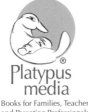

Platypus Media, LLC
725 Eighth Street, SE
Washington, DC 20003
Tel: 202-546-1674
Toll free: 877-752-8977
Fax: 202-546-2356
Website: PlatypusMedia.com
Email: Info@PlatypusMedia.com

Books for Families, Teachers
and Parenting Professionals

To request a catalog, permission to reprint, or bulk purchasing information, please contact us at the address above.

Health care professionals, government agencies, and non-profit organizations can receive a bulk discount for quantity orders.

10 9 8 7 6 5 4 3 2 1

All rights reserved. No part of this publication may be reproduced or transmitted in any form or by any means, electronic or mechanical, including photocopy, recording, or any information storage and retrieval system, without permission in writing from the publisher.

Printed in the United States of America.

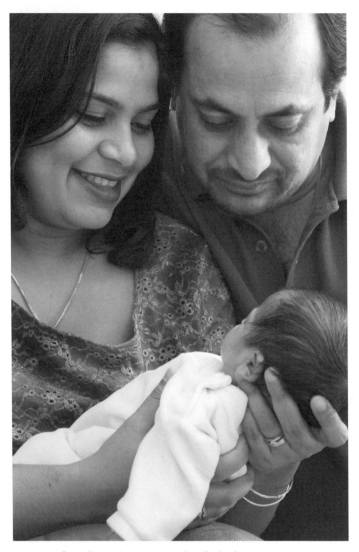

Breastfeeding is a wonderful chance to provide the best for your baby, your partner and your family. It is not only the most perfect and most natural food available, but it also promotes bonding, protects both mom and baby from a wide range of illnesses, and is the most direct route to a smart and happy child.

Table of Contents

Why Is Breastfeeding So Important?

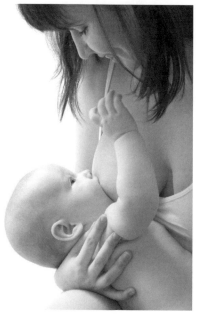

Humans have been breastfeeding for at least 400,000 years because breastmilk is the optimal food for growing babies. It is important for you as a father to know the benefits for your baby and for the whole family as you influence the first of many decisions in your child's life. You will become a teacher, a coach, a supporter, and a role model.

Breastfeeding is not only about mom and baby. **Among the greatest factors that determine whether or not a mother will breastfeed is the support of the baby's father.** Research has shown that when fathers were completely supportive, mothers working outside the home breastfed 98.1 percent of the time, but when fathers were indifferent, mothers only breastfed 26.9 percent of the time. If you want your family to have all the benefits of breastfeeding, it is crucial that you strongly encourage your baby's mother to breastfeed.

"You new dads shouldn't feel left out when it comes to baby's mealtime. Breastfeeding is one of the healthiest things that can be done for your newborn."
Dean Edell, MD, host of the Dr. Dean Edell Show

Fathering without Feeding

"Every baby needs a non-nutritive parent. That's the father."

> Ruth A. Lawrence, MD, Author, *Breastfeeding: A Guide for the Medical Profession*

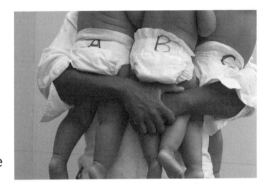

Dads might feel excluded from mom and baby's breastfeeding relationship during the first few months, but it is important to keep in mind that a father is the first person to show his baby that feeding does not equal love. Humans are born more helpless than any other animal, and they need to spend more time as children learning from their environment. A father's unique relationship with his baby is an important element in a child's development from early infancy.

Fathers encourage their children to use new words, to engage in games, and to use their arms and legs in play. They can bathe them, cosleep with them at night, wear them on outings, feed their baby mom's pumped breastmilk when mom is away, and just hang out together. While breastfeeding does create a strong tie between mother and baby, there is no shortage of rewarding work for dads. Breastfeeding is only temporary, but the benefits are long-lasting, and in no time at all, your child will be exploring the world outside his mother's arms.

What the Doctors Recommend

"A millionaire's baby fed with commercial baby milk has a poorer diet than the poorest family's baby who is breastfed."

– World Health Organization, 1997

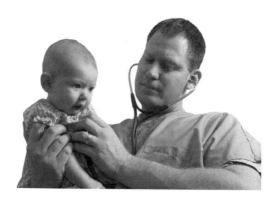

The American Academy of Pediatrics (80,000 physicians who work with babies and children) advises that babies should be fed breastmilk exclusively for the first six months of life. During this time, no water, juice or foods should be given.

After six months, breastfeeding should continue in addition to complementary foods for at least a year. Mom should continue breastfeeding until she and her baby decide they are ready to wean. All the experts agree that breastmilk is good for baby, not just as food, but as a powerful protection against ailments such as allergies and ear infections, and can even reduce the chances of Sudden Infant Death Syndrome (SIDS) as well as a number of other diseases.

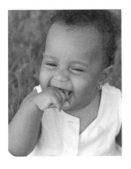

Why You Want Your Baby Breastfed

Babies that are fed breastmilk are happier and healthier than formula-fed babies. Why?

Breastfeeding:

- Gives antibodies from mom to baby to boost baby's immune system;
- Helps bond mother and child;
- Provides food that is easily digestible for baby;
- Confers passive immunity;
- Helps protect against measles, chicken pox, and other contagious diseases;
- Promotes normal growth and neurological development;
- Prevents hypothermia in the newborn;
- Provides partial protection against necrotizing enterocolitis, a gastrointestinal disease that often affects premature infants;
- Provides significant protection against bacteremia, meningitis, and neonatal sepsis;
- Promotes proper tooth, jaw, and visual development;
- Adapts to meet the needs of premature and low birth weight babies;
- Helps develop a baby's cognitive ability.

Liquid Gold for the Newborn

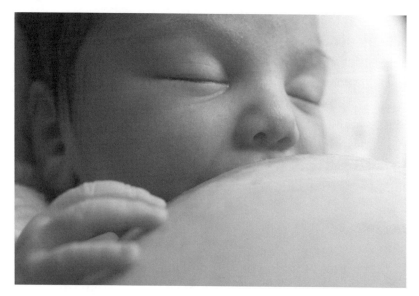

In the first few days of a baby's life, mom produces a substance that is rich in proteins called colostrum. Its white blood cells protect baby from infections and its antibodies protect baby's digestive system. It also stimulates a baby's first bowel movements. If babies do not have colostrum during their first three days of life, their immune system does not enjoy these benefits. It is truly a once-in-a-lifetime opportunity.

"Human milk is often called 'liquid gold.' This reflects the golden hue of colostrum, a mother's first milk, but more importantly, the value of the irreproducible nutrients, antibodies, and growth factors babies receive with each nursing."

Sharing the Health: Mothers' Milk Bank of New England 2008

Benefits for Life

In addition to its benefits during infancy, breastfeeding has advantages that last throughout childhood and into adulthood. Breastfed babies become physically healthy children and adults. They are less likely to suffer from infectious illnesses such as ear

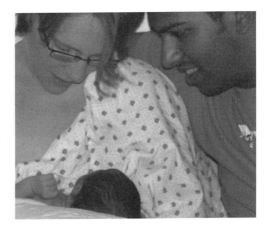

infections, respiratory tract infections, and meningitis, and have lower rates of Crohn's disease, ulcerative colitis, asthma, eczema, and juvenile diabetes. The benefits extend into adulthood, when those who were breastfed have lower rates of atherosclerosis, breast cancer, adult diabetes, blood infections, urinary tract infections, multiple sclerosis, and osteoporosis.

Many studies have shown a connection between breastfeeding and cognitive development. Babies who are breastfed for at least eight months have a lower risk of developing language impairments; higher IQs at ages eight and nine; better reading comprehension, mathematical skills and scholastic ability from ages 10 to 13; and higher academic achievements in high school.

"Bottle-fed babies are twice as likely to have crooked teeth because rubber nipples do not conform to the unique shape of babies' mouths, as breasts do. Breastfeeding is baby's first workout."

Brian Palmer, DDS, "The Influence of Breastfeeding on the Development of the Oral Cavity"

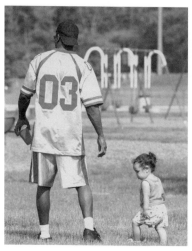

The benefits of breastfeeding are not only physical, but psychological as well, with breastfed babies demonstrating lower levels of stress, anxiety, depression, schizophrenia, and more.

Increased breastfeeding can also reduce your child's chances of becoming obese later in life. Children who are breastfed exclusively during their first six months are 22 percent less likely to become obese between the ages of 9 and 14. This percentage goes up with each additional month that your child is breastfed. Breastfeeding beyond a child's first birthday is even better, decreasing a baby's risk of obesity by 72 percent. Breastfed babies have higher levels of leptin, a hormone that helps to regulate appetite. They are better able to program themselves to stop eating when they are full, learning to self-regulate their caloric intake over time. Bottle-fed babies are often overfed because parents want the bottle's entire contents to be consumed. This overfeeding can increase the number of permanent fat cells. In addition, babies who are fed formula during the critical early weeks experience changes in their pancreatic islets, which lead to overproduction of insulin and adult obesity. Formula is made with sucrose, essentially white table sugar, which is much sweeter than lactose, the sugar found in breastmilk. Therefore, formula-fed babies typically develop an unnatural affinity for sweet, fatty foods.

Is Formula Really So Bad?

It was never the plan for infant formula to be as widely consumed as it is today. It was originally developed in the 1800s to feed orphan babies who otherwise would have starved. While formula is better for babies than regular milk, it does not contain all of the significant ingredients that make up breastmilk: white blood cells, active digestive enzymes, immunoglobulins, and lactose. It does, however, contain many ingredients that are difficult for the baby's stomach to break down. Breastmilk is a living biological fluid; formula is not.

Donor milk from a human breastmilk bank is readily available in the U.S. as a prescription item and is a better choice than infant formula.

Infant formula is not only inferior nutritionally, but it can also be dangerous. The National Alliance for Breastfeeding Advocacy (NABA) keeps a list of formula recalls available at http://www.naba-breastfeeding.org/images/Recalls.pdf. There have been many instances where infant formula was recalled because it posed a serious threat to the health of babies who consumed it. Recalls of both powdered and ready-to-feed formulas are often issued for reasons such as deficient or excessive vitamin levels, glass particles, curdling, bacterial or chemical contamination, and salmonella contamination. Sadly, this information rarely gets to the consumers. The only way to guarantee that your baby is not exposed to these dangers is to breastfeed exclusively.

Why Is Breastmilk a Much Healthier Choice?

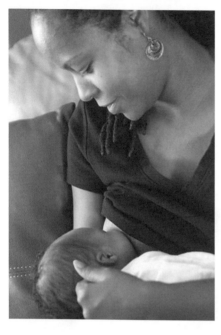

Compared to breastfed babies, formula-fed babies are:

TWICE as likely to die from any cause in the first six weeks of life;

TWO TO FIVE times more likely to die of Sudden Infant Death Syndrome (SIDS);

TWICE as likely to suffer from diarrhea, the leading cause of death for infants;

FIVE times more likely to develop urinary tract infections;

TWICE as likely to develop juvenile-onset insulin-dependent (type 1) diabetes;

TWICE as likely to suffer from inner-ear infection;

MORE likely to have cavities and require braces in later life;

MORE likely to have a higher risk of childhood and adolescent obesity;

MORE likely to suffer from some forms of cancer (e.g., Hodgkin's disease and childhood leukemia);

MORE likely to have allergies;

AND... more likely to have lower IQs.

A Happier, Healthier Mom

Breastfeeding is not only beneficial for baby, but also for mom. Mothers who breastfeed enjoy a quicker recovery from childbirth with less risk of bleeding, and are more likely to return to their pre-pregnancy weight. Breastfeeding can burn between 350-500 extra calories per day, the equivalent of running three to five miles. In addition, mother's uterus will return more quickly to its normal size.

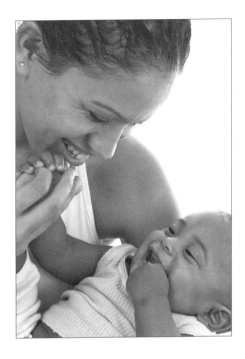

Mom's benefits, like baby's, are also long-term. Women who have breastfed are less likely to develop ovarian and pre-menopausal breast cancers. A woman who breastfeeds for 24 months cuts her risk of breast cancer in half.

Breastfeeding mothers are also reported to be more confident and less anxious than bottle-feeding mothers. This is because breastfeeding produces two great hormones, oxytocin and prolactin, whose side effects leave mom feeling euphoric and calm. Scientists believe that prolactin is crucial to a mother's acceptance of her young.

When Breastfeeding Is Not Advised

Contraindications to breastfeeding are extremely rare, and under ordinary circumstances, infants should always be breastfed. Here are some exceptions, though you should always review individual situations with your health care provider and lactation consultant.

Reason	Effect on Baby	Expert Advice
Toxemia/Pre-eclampsia	Some medications used to treat mom could be harmful to baby, so breastfeeding should be delayed until treatment is completed.	Milk should be discarded until treatment is complete and then breastfeeding can be initiated.
Amphetamines, speed, methadrine, ritalin	These make baby agitated, spoil his appetite, and interfere with normal growth and development.	Mom should not breastfeed.
Cocaine, crack	These drugs actually poison baby.	Mom should not breastfeed.
AIDS and HIV Positive	Although infected lymphocytes do contain the virus and may transmit the disease, baby still needs the advantages of breastmilk.	Health care professionals can work with mom to obtain banked breastmilk or to sterilize mom's pumped milk.
Breast cancer	Chemotherapy can poison baby.	Mom should not breastfeed during treatment, but cancer survivors, including breast cancer survivors, can breastfeed.
Galactosemia	If baby has galactosemia – though it only occurs in one in every 60,000 to 80,000 births – he or she cannot metabolize lactose, a milk sugar found in breastmilk.	Mom should not breastfeed.

Information Regarding Medications
The vast majority of over the counter and prescription medications can be used by breastfeeding moms. There are only a few instances when a single medication or class of medications are potentially harmful while breastfeeding. The books by Thomas Hale, PhD and Dr. Stephen Buescher, listed on page 34, will provide you with the most current and accurate information on medication use during breastfeeding. For more information, visit the Drugs and Lactation Database by the U.S. National Library of Medicine at http://toxnet.nlm.nih.gov/cgi-bin/sis/htmlgen?LACT.

You Should Still Breastfeed Even If...

Reason	Effect on Baby	Expert Advice
You have shingles, chicken pox, or varicella	Breastmilk is a source of antibodies. If both mom and baby are infected, they should be isolated together and breastfeeding should continue.	If mom has lesions, and baby is healthy, mom should be isolated, but can pump milk for baby to drink. As soon as lesions heal, mom and baby can be reunited and breastfeeding reinstated.
You have Hepatitis A, B, or C	Though all forms of the Hepatitis virus are found in breastmilk, only Hepatitis B is infectious. Baby can continue to nurse.	Babies born to mothers who have Hepatitis B should be immunized with a vaccine and Hepatitis B immuno-globulin within the first 12 hours of life. There is no reason to discontinue breastfeeding.
You have a common cold, flu, or bronchitis	Baby needs immunity conferred by breastmilk, as well as continuing attachment to mom even though she is ill. There is no reason to discontinue breastfeeding.	Baby has been exposed to her germs already, and through breastfeeding, is also receiving antibodies to protect him from disease-causing germs.
You are taking ACE Inhibitors	Baby is likely to develop low blood pressure.	Caution should be taken during the first two weeks after delivery, but after that, breastfeeding is fine.
You are taking oral steroids	These inhibit baby's bone growth. Breast-feeding may continue, but dosage may need to be adjusted in order to minimize effects on baby.	If these are used chronically, Mom should consult a physician concerning her dosage.

If you have questions or concerns about breastfeeding, contact a lactation consultant. Visit http://www.ILCA.org and click on "Find a Lactation Consultant."

You Should Still Breastfeed Even If...

Reason	Effect on Baby	Expert Advice
You are taking statins or other cholesterol lowering medication.	These lower baby's cholesterol and inhibit baby's growth.	Mom should take a break from these drugs. One-to-two years of not taking these medications does not affect the long-term outcome.
You do "not have enough milk"*	Baby seems hungry all the time.	While this is a common concern, moms usually have plenty of milk. Extending feeding time and pumping may increase milk. A lactation consultant can suggest ways to increase milk supply through herbs, medication, feeding strategies, etc.
You have mastitis	Mom may feel awful but baby will be fine nursing.	Antibiotics can clear this up. Frequent nursing can help clear the breast ducts.
You have sore breasts	Breast soreness can be uncomfortable when breasts are engorged.	Nurse often, don't skip feedings (even at night), allow baby to finish the first breast before offering the other side. Check with a lactation consultant to ensure that you have a correct latch and positioning. Stand under the water of a warm shower. Apply cabbage leaf compresses to the breasts to relieve engorgement.
You smoke	Baby will be affected by the harmful effects of tobacco and other chemicals in the mother's bloodstream.	Although nicotine can be found in the breastmilk of mothers who smoke, and mothers should always try to quit, it is better to give a baby this breastmilk than to give him formula.
Your baby is ill with anything besides galactosemia, including gastrointestinal infections and diarrhea	Baby needs the immunity boost only breastmilk can provide in order to build a strong and robust immune system.	Mom should keep breastfeeding in order to provide baby with health benefits that will last a lifetime.

*During the first week, frequent nursing should result in one wet diaper on day one, two on day two, three on day three, four on day four, five on day five, and six on day six. After the first week, babies should have at least five wet diapers each twenty-four hour period, and at least two bowel movements, after nursing at least eight times. You can refer to the Diaper Diary by LactNews at http://www.lactnews.com/englishdd.html. Seek the advice of a health care professional immediately if you are concerned about your baby's well-being.

How Does Breastfeeding Really Work?

Breastfeeding is a mechanical process powered by hormones. The baby's stimulation of nerves in the nipples causes mom's pituitary gland to release two hormones: prolactin, which stimulates the cells to produce milk, and oxytocin, which causes the milk-producing cells to contract and push the milk out through the ducts and into the baby's mouth. This is called the let-down reflex.

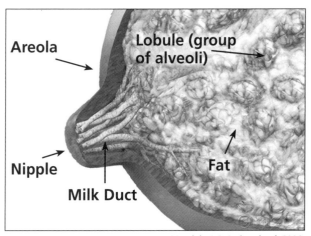

Areola

Lobule (group of alveoli)

Nipple

Fat

Milk Duct

©Medela AG, Switzerland, 2006

Milk is produced in the alveolus, and travels through the milk ducts, which expand and drain out through the nipple. Milk is stored in these ducts, and mothers continue making milk between feedings. While the baby is nursing, the mother's breasts are stimulated to make more milk than they do between feedings, so the more often she breastfeeds, the more milk she will produce. When a baby suckles at the nipple, stimulating oxytocin release, Mom's nipple elongates to about twice its normal length. The oxytocin causes a contraction of the milk ducts, moving the milk down toward the nipple. During the first few months, moms may feel pressure or tingling during milk ejection.

Can We Get Pregnant While Breastfeeding?

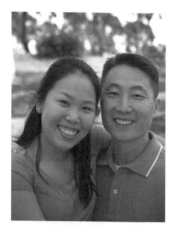

Sex will not be satisfactory if you are both worried about getting pregnant again. The return to fertility is usually delayed in breastfeeding women because of lowered estrogen levels, but the length of delay varies from woman to woman. Approximately 80 percent of breastfeeding women are not fertile until the return of their period, which means that one in five breastfeeding women can conceive even if they are not yet menstruating again. If you are unwilling to take that chance, various forms of contraception are available. Hormonal birth control has shown to deplete milk supply in many mothers; however, the contraceptive ring (which has very low hormone levels) and the diaphram are, along with condoms, both good options. Talk with your physician or your partner's gynecologist to explore the best options.

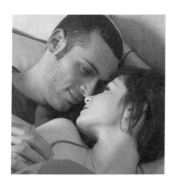

Sex and the Breastfeeding Woman

New mothers are more often than not less interested in sex after having a baby and throughout breastfeeding due to a number of physical and psychological factors. Sometimes fathers feel the same way. Many women experience a great deal of fatigue with a new baby, and you probably will as well. Weakened abdominal muscles, as well as larger hips, thighs, and breasts can make mothers feel uncomfortable or "unsexy" as they adjust to the changes in their body shape. Many women also experience pain during sex after having a baby, and this can discourage them from wanting to be intimate. There is usually a great deal of anxiety, stress, and sometimes even depression accompanying a new baby, which may have an impact on your desire for intimacy as a couple. What many don't know is that experiencing these problems is completely natural.

Did you know:
- There is some disturbance in almost all sexual relationships after birth, and most couples have fears about making love;
- Most couples do not enjoy intercourse for at least two months after birth; most, however, say that their sexual desire returned to prepregnancy level, or even increased, after a while;
- It is common for milk to spurt from a breastfeeding woman's nipples during sex;
- Many women feel more sexually confident after birth from a new sense of femininity, maturity and awareness of their bodies; and
- Breastfeeding women, fueled by the hormones oxytocin and prolactin, usually have strong feelings of peace and happiness.

Breastfeeding causes hormonal fluctuations that might alter a woman's interest in sex while she is still breastfeeding. Estrogen and progesterone, two reproductive hormones, increase during pregnancy and then drop sharply after childbirth. 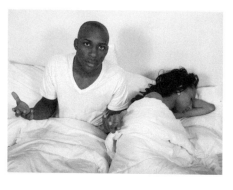 The presence of these hormones increases a woman's libido, and the lack of them can partially account for a woman's decreased sexual drive after birth. She might also experience decreased vaginal lubrication. Breastfeeding greatly delays the return to normal levels of these hormones, and can therefore also delay the return of a desire for intimacy.

Another important factor in postnatal intimacy is exhaustion. A new baby is more work than you might expect and tiredness is the most common cause for abstinence in the first few weeks or months after birth. Many couples report that their interest in sex resumed when they had time for a good night's sleep.

A recent study found that over 40 percent of women experienced pain during their first postnatal intercourse, largely because of small cuts and tears from birth or from a lack of lubrication. Keep in mind that the wounds will heal, and other forms of lubrication are available, such as KY and Aquaglide, until moisture levels are back to normal.

Try This...

Many women report an increased interest in sex (even higher than before birth) after they begin ovulating and their hormone levels return to normal. There are several things that you can do, both inside and outside of the bedroom, to help you and your partner adjust to enjoyable intimacy after having a baby:

- Try to talk to, touch, and support your partner as much as possible. This can reduce stress as well as bring you closer together;
- Take care of yourself. Make sure you eat well and get enough sleep to ease stress, as well as make time to spend with friends and family;
- Plan for sex. Though you might be used to more spontaneous intimacy, this often becomes extremely difficult, if not impossible, after a baby is born;
- Help your partner relax before intimacy. She may feel stressed, nervous about her physical appearance, or worried about pain. Do all that you can to calm her and reassure her;
- Help ease pain during intercourse. Find positions that are comfortable for both of you, stock up on lubricant to ease dryness and tenderness, and remember to take your time;
- Keep an open mind while adjusting. Look for information that might help, be open to exploring other ways to be intimate, and remember to always communicate with your partner;
- Help ease the strain at home by cooking dinner or taking your child(ren) for a walk while she cooks. Make sure she has as much control over her own life as possible. Give her some "time out" by looking after the baby.

Be patient and continue to have a positive attitude.

What If I Am Separated from My Baby's Mom?

Even if you are separated from your baby's mother, you are still the father of your child, with all of the benefits and responsibilities that the role entails. The exclusive mom-baby breastfeeding relationship may appear to threaten a father's parenting time with his child after a separation. The first few weeks might be particularly difficult since it is best for babies

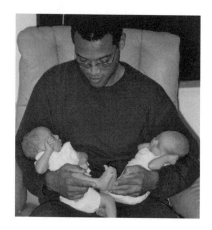

to feed directly at the breast and they need to spend most of their time with mom. But later on, you can feed your baby mom's pumped breastmilk from a bottle. You can also be aware of your baby's developmental stages, as you put his or her needs above your own.

As a matter of public policy, social service agencies encourage children to have close relationships with both parents. In custody disputes, courts may recognize that breastfeeding is best for the baby, but will not sacrifice the father-child bond to allow the mother to continue breastfeeding. It is rare for a court to postpone overnight visitation past the age of two. Fathers who are negotiating a divorce settlement should prepare a specific parenting time schedule if they are trying to arrange visitation with their children. The courts usually figure the maximum rather than the minimum time that babies tolerate being separated from their nursing mothers.

Can We Sleep with Our Baby?

"Many children are less physically and emotionally healthy than they could be. The current epidemic of childhood obesity suggests that children are overfed but probably undernourished... What is a successful child? A child who's happy, well adjusted, and morally grounded... a successful child is an attached child – connected not just to family, but to the world beyond."

William Sears, MD and Martha Sears, RN
The Successful Child

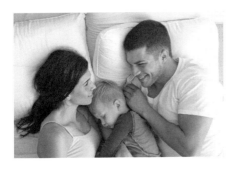

Absolutely. Sleeping with your baby is an excellent opportunity for you to bond with your baby, and makes it easier for your baby's mother to breastfeed during the night. One of the most important things a father can do for his new baby is to hold him. The skin-to-skin contact helps regulate the baby's body temperature and rhythmic functions, such as heartbeat and breathing. At birth, the human baby's brain capacity is not yet fully developed, making him helpless for the first year. You and mom are the main providers of the human contact that your baby needs to develop into a healthy, intelligent and confident adult. You can help stimulate your baby's growing brain by constantly touching and talking to him. In addition, the rate of SIDS (Sudden Infant Death Syndrome) is possibly reduced in babies who sleep with their parents because their sleep cycle is regulated, and you and mom can keep watch over your baby. The family bed gives both parents more opportunities to read, sing, cuddle, hold and play with their infant, while providing the critical role of being "a newborn surveillance system."

If You Want to Sleep with Your Baby

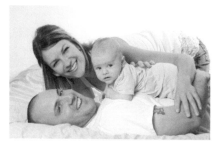

Sleeping with a baby can be a wonderful, nurturing, and protective experience. However, it needs to be done safely so that your baby does not become tangled in bedding or rolled upon by a parent, sibling, or pet. Here are some guidelines for sleeping safely with your baby:

1. The mattress must be firm. If your mattress is squishy, put a board under it so that your baby does not sink into it while sleeping. Never put your baby on a waterbed.

2. Do not sleep with your baby if you or your partner smokes tobacco or marijuana, even if you only smoke outside the house. SIDS research shows that the residue from smoking can be a cause of Sudden Infant Death Syndrome.

3. Humans are programmed to be aware of their baby even while sleeping; however, alcohol, sedatives, or medications can lessen that ability. Drinking or taking drugs will impair responsiveness to your baby's needs, so don't sleep with your baby if you use any substances that cause altered consciousness.

4. You may be tempted to bring toys for the baby into your bed. Don't. Stuffed toys and pillows can suffocate a sleeping baby.

5. Do not allow other children into bed with baby. Do not allow pets in the bed.

Frequently Asked Questions

Frequently Asked Questions

How Often Should Mom Breastfeed?

In the early weeks, mother should try to breastfeed on both breasts each feeding. She should breastfeed on the first breast until the baby comes off by himself, usually after about 15 to 20 minutes, and then offer the other side. Babies know how much milk they need.

Every baby is different, so the clock should not determine when mom breastfeeds again. Your baby will need to breastfeed whenever he shows signs of hunger, for example, squirming, sucking his fists, licking his lips or rooting (turning his head to look for the breast). You can help look for these signs in your baby. Healthy, full-term babies may breastfeed as often as every hour or as infrequently as every four hours. Many babies also "cluster feed" in the evening before their bedtime; they nurse almost constantly for several hours, not only taking both sides, but going back and forth a few times before they are finished. Babies often cluster feed just to find comfort and to calm down, not because their mother is not making enough milk.

Does Breastfeeding Hurt?

It does not and should not hurt. If it does, there's something wrong with the way the baby is attached, or latched onto, the breast. The nipples might be tender during the first couple of feeds, but aside from that, breastfeeding should not be painful. If it is, you should talk to a La Leche League leader or lactation consultant.

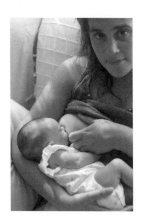

How Do I Know If My Baby Is Getting Enough Milk?

During the first week, you can tell by looking at your baby's poop. At first, it should be black and sticky, but by the third or fourth day, it should be greenish, and then will gradually turn into a light yellow. If it is light in color by day three, your baby is probably getting enough milk. Your baby should have two wet diapers by the second day, three on the third, and four on the fourth. By the end of the first week, babies should have at least six to eight

---

wet diapers a day and two to three dirty ones. Breastfed babies' poop is loose and runny and looks a lot like mustard. This is not diarrhea. Breastfed babies rarely get diarrhea, and if they do, it is foul-smelling and watery. If your baby is content and nurses when he needs to, he is probably getting enough milk. You can also refer to the Diaper Diary at http://www.lactnews.com/englishdd.html.

What If My Baby's Mom Can't Breastfeed?

Mothers and babies are almost always physically able to breastfeed; it is very unusual not to be able to. Given support and correct information, at least 97 percent of women can breastfeed successfully and produce enough milk for their babies not just to grow, but to thrive. The usual responses for why some women don't breastfeed include the following: "I tried breastfeeding, but it didn't work; it was painful; I didn't have enough milk; I leaked too much; or my baby didn't seem satisfied." A large problem is the lack of education in the management of breastfeeding, such as knowing how to position the baby. You can often overcome these barriers with the help of a La Leche League Leader or lactation consultant.

How Long Should Mom Breastfeed?

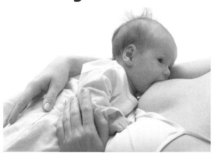

No one rule works best here. In a number of countries – from Norway to Iran to Togo – women commonly breastfeed their babies for well over a year. There is no documented figure worldwide, but several experts estimate the average to be around three years. Weaning is a developmental stage and babies wean when they are ready. The most important thing to remember is that your baby should not consume water, juice or foods during the first six months. After six months, when babies begin eating more solid foods, it is natural to let them decide if they want to nurse less or not. Some babies nurse along with eating solids for two years or more, all the while continuing to reap the health benefits from nursing.

Frequently Asked Questions *continued*

Breastfeeding is a mutual relationship between mom and baby. Some babies lose interest, but if both enjoy the relationship, there is no reason not to continue.

> Parenthood brings supreme meaning and joy to our lives. When a mother suckles her child, she gives expression to that joy. When a mother offers her breast, she offers her time, her warmth, herself. The baby takes in food; and while it appears that something is being removed from one and given to the other, it is actually love that is being exchanged.

Is There Anything Mom Can't Eat?

There are no particular foods that are prohibited for breastfeeding mothers. Advice varies between different cultures. In Italy, mothers are often told not to eat garlic, cauliflower, lentils or red peppers, and in India, most mothers eat all of the above and breastfeed happily. In fact, in some parts of India, it is believed that garlic actually helps a mother breastfeed successfully. As long as mom maintains a well-balanced and nutritious diet, everything should be fine. Eating a variety of fresh, healthy foods is always good. She should avoid any foods she or dad are sensitive to while the baby is quite young, particularly if either side of the family is prone to allergies. Some very sensitive babies react to specific foods in their mother's diet. Common culprits are cow's milk products, wheat, corn, and tomatoes. If you notice that your baby is fussy, experiment with eliminating certain foods from mom's diet.

What about Breastfeeding and Nipple Piercings?

Body piercing is no longer just for ear lobes; women have increasingly pierced lips, navels, and nipples. Fortunately, nipple piercing is compatible with breastfeeding, as long as the piercing is no longer fresh. While in some instances piercing could increase milk flow (not production), in others, a piercing could cause scar tissue and close a duct. Mom should have enough milk even with a closed duct, but she may have some engorgement as that duct produces milk but does

---

Frequently Asked Questions *continued*

not have an outlet. Mom should remove the jewelry either before each feeding or for the entire nursing period, as it can cause choking or discomfort for both mom and the baby, and the baby might have difficulty latching onto the nipple if jewelry is in the way. If she doesn't have a piercing already but is interested in getting one, it is best to wait until her baby is weaned.

What about Breastfeeding and Implants?

Whether or not a woman with implants will be able to breastfeed depends on her particular surgery; she should consult her doctor about the procedure that was used before attempting to breastfeed. While there is no evidence that silicone from silicone implants leaks into a mother's breastmilk, nerve damage on her breasts might prevent her from being able to trigger or release milk. Incisions made under the fold of the breast or through the armpit shouldn't cause any trouble, but the method of making a "smile" around the areola could disturb the milk ducts that transfer milk from the breast lobe to the nipples. Yet, many women with implants are still able to breastfeed, either fully or partially. A Supplemental Nursing System can be a useful tool in supporting the breastfeeding mom who is unable to produce sufficient milk. Your doctor can monitor whether or not your baby is getting enough to eat, and La Leche League International and a lactation consultant are good resources for more help and information.

What about Alcohol and Breastfeeding?

The risks of consuming alcohol while breastfeeding are not as concrete as those while pregnant. Generally, the effects of alcohol on the breastfeeding baby are directly related to the amount the mother drinks. If she drinks occasionally or limits her consumption to one drink or less per day, the amount of alcohol her baby receives has not been proven to be harmful.

The American Academy of Pediatrics Committee on Drugs considers limited alcohol acceptable during breastfeeding. It lists possible side effects if consumed in large amounts, including drowsiness, deep sleep, weakness, and abnormal weight gain in the infant, and the possibility of decreased milk-ejection reflex in the mother. One rule of thumb is to wait one hour per each drink before breastfeeding, in order to allow mom's body to metabolize the alcohol. However, many mothers do enjoy a glass of wine with dinner and nurse at the same time, without waiting one hour. It is important to eat while consuming the alcohol.

Will Breastfeeding Make Her Breasts Sag?

Despite the common myth, breastfeeding does not make breasts sag. In a recent study presented at the American Society of Plastic Surgeons, there was no difference in the degree of ptosis (or sagging) between women who breastfed and those who didn't. It is actually the processes of pregnancy, heredity, aging, and, of course, gravity that lead to drooping breasts. Pregnant and breastfeeding moms and their partners often enjoy the extra fullness that breastfeeding and pregnancy provide.

Will Mom Run Out of Milk?

Not usually. Baby needs to be fed very frequently during the first few weeks, and mother's milk production will adjust according to her baby's changing needs. Moms produce milk as long as their baby is nursing. Insufficient milk intake is commonly caused by infrequent nursing, limited time at the breast, or the use of pacifiers and/or poor latching. There are a handful of prescription drugs, as well as a number of galactogogues (foods that increase milk supply) that moms can use to boost breastmilk volume. In addition, a Supplemental Nursing System can help mom nurse while either supplementing or building up her own breastmilk supply. If low milk supply is an issue, contact La Leche League International or a lactation consultant.

Won't It Be Embarrassing in Public?

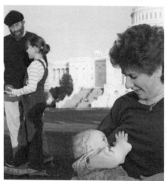

For some men and women, there can be embarrassment associated with breastfeeding in public. You should be proud and delighted that your baby is getting the best start in life. You can help mom feel more comfortable, hold the baby while she situates herself, and take on any strangers' questions.

There is no reason for a mother to fully expose her breasts in order to feed her

---

Frequently Asked Questions *continued*

baby in public; it is easy for her to breastfeed discreetly if she wears the right clothes. A loose-fitting top that lifts or can be unbuttoned from the waist up will let her feed your baby without exposing her breast because the baby will cover her nipple and lower breast. You can also buy her special nursing bathing suits, dresses, or shirts with hidden slits and panels. It is completely legal to breastfeed in public. You can help her practice being discreet before you go out in public, or she can practice in front of a mirror.

Can Adults Drink Breastmilk?

Technically, yes. Human milk is best for human babies, just as whale milk is best for whale babies, but breastmilk can be a first food, a complementary food, and even a sole source of nourishment for adults in times of famine. All humans, not only babies, can drink breastmilk. It has been sought after in illness and war, and is sometimes used after surgeries to build the immune system. The Human Milk Banking Association of North America (www.hmbana.org) collects, screens, processes and distributes human milk for adult medical purposes.

Why Don't Some Women Breastfeed?

Breastfeeding rates in many countries, including in the U.S. and the United Kingdom, are catastrophically low. Younger women in particular are less likely to breastfeed, but the biggest gap is socio-economic. The poorer a woman is, the less likely she is to breastfeed. Watching others in a family or community was traditionally the way in which many learned to breastfeed, but now, many families have gone a generation or two without breastfeeding; young mothers need to find someone else to teach them.

The producers of infant formula are one of the biggest reasons for this development. As they are spending billions of dollars promoting their product over breastmilk, women are becoming confused about breastfeeding. While new international laws are being implemented to prevent companies from advertising infant-formula directly to mothers (through give-aways in hospitals and ads in mothering magazines), there is a long way to go.

Breastfeeding Facts for Fathers

Frequently Asked Questions *continued*

While breastfeeding initiation rates have now risen to 74 percent, exclusive breastfeeding during the first three months after birth is just 31 percent, decreasing to just 11 percent for the first six months. Many women want to breastfeed, but they give up soon after starting because they don't know enough about keeping up with it. When a woman wants to breastfeed but is experiencing difficulties, she needs a social support network, which is often missing.

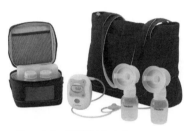

Copyright ©2008 Medela Inc.

What Should We Do When My Baby's Mom Returns to Work?

Breastfeeding mothers can return to work with the proper information and planning. Since few women are with their babies around the clock, pumping can become a daily routine like flossing, commuting, or shaving. Luckily, breast pumping can simulate the baby's sucking and trigger Mom's brain to make more milk.

Once a mom determines the amount of breastmilk her child needs, she can regulate her milk supply by adjusting her pumping schedule.

Laws in many states call for mothers who are employed to receive breaks, flextime, and job-sharing arrangements that promote breastfeeding. Pumping breaks are often covered by law and it is the practice in many family-oriented companies. The U.S. Department of Health and Human Services (HHS) also offers a free kit with booklets for the human resources department, the employer and the employee; it is called *The Business Case for Breastfeeding* and can be ordered at 1-800-AskHRSA.

The Surgeon General's Office states that breastfeeding is the normal way to feed infants, and mothers should be free to feed their babies in the places where they live and work.

The best support for a breastfeeding mother is often her partner, so be there for her and you will get a healthy family in return.

Notes and Sources

4)   Littman, Heidi. "The Decision to Breastfeed: The Importance of Fathers' Approval." *Clinical Pediatrics* 33 (1994): 214-19. Available at http://cpj.sagepub.com/cgi/content/abstract/33/4/214.
       Riordan, Jan. *Breastfeeding and Human Lactation*. Sudbury, MA: Jones and Bartlett Publishers, Inc., 2005.

6)   Gupta, Arun. "Why ensure exclusive breastfeeding for all babies?" OneWorld: 2004. Available at http://us.oneworld.net/node/91300
       Hale, Thomas. *Medications and Mothers' Milk*. Amarillo, Texas: Hale Publishing, L.P. 12th Edition, 2006.

7)   Baumslag, N., and D.L. Michels. *Milk, Money and Madness: The Culture and Politics of Breastfeeding*. Wesport, CT: Bergin & Garvey, 1995.

8)   "Breastfeeding and the Use of Human Milk." American Academy of Pediatrics 6 (2005): 1035-1039.

9-10) United States Breastfeeding Committee. *Benefits of Breastfeeding* [issue paper]. Raleigh, NC: United States Breastfeeding Committee; 2002. Available at http://www.usbreastfeeding.org/Issue-Papers/Benefits.pdf
       Chudler, Eric H. "Brain Development." University of Washington: 1996-2008. Available at http://faculty.washington.edu/chudler/dev.html
       Michels, Dia. "Breastfeeding – An Obesity Prophylactic." *Mothering Magazine*. July / August 2003.
       INFACT Canada. "Health Protection and Health Care in Canada." February 13, 2002. Available at http://www.infactcanada.ca/news_releases_Romanow.htm
       La Leche League International. "Born to Learn: Selected Bibliography 2001." Available at http://www.llli.org/cbi/bibborn.html.

11-12) Baby Milk Action. "The UK Law: Briefing Paper." Available at http://www.babymilkaction.org/pages/uklaw.html

13)   Hale, Dr. Thomas W. *A Medication Guide for Breastfeeding Moms*. Amarillo, Texas: Pharmasoft Medical Publishing, 2005.
       "Hormone Involved in Reproduction May Have Role in the Maintenance of Relationships." 1999. Available at www.oxytocin.org/oxytoc/
       "Why Should You Breastfeed Your Baby?" National Women's Health Information Center. U.S. Department of Health and Human Services. Available at www.4woman.gov/Breastfeeding

14-16) Buescher, E. Stephen. *Breastfeeding and Diseases: A Reference Guide*. Amarillo, Texas: Hale Publishing, L.P., 2008.
       Hale, Thomas. *Medications and Mothers' Milk*. Amarillo, Texas: Hale Publishing, L.P.; 12th Edition, 2006.

17)   Baumslag, N., and D.L. Michels. *Milk, Money and Madness: The Culture and Politics of Breastfeeding*. Westport, CT: Bergin & Garvey, 1995.

Notes and Sources *continued*

18-21)   "Sex After Childbirth." Available at http://www.ninemonths.com.au/
         adjusting-to-parenthood/sex-after-childbirth.html
23-24)   McKenna, James J. *Sleeping With Your Baby: A Parent's Guide to
         Cosleeping*. Washington, DC: Platypus Media, 2007.
         Sears, W., MD. "Safe Co-Sleeping." Available at www.iparenting.com/
         sears/columns/co-sleep.htm
25-30)   Baumslag, N., and D.L. Michels. *Milk, Money and Madness: The Culture
         and Politics of Breastfeeding*. Westport, CT: Bergin & Garvey, 1995.
31)   Bromberg Bar-Yam, N. "What Every Breastfeeding Employee Should
         Know." *Breastfeeding Annual International*. Ed. D.L. Michels.
         Washington, DC: Platypus Media, 2001: 72-81.

Photo Credits

Front Cover	Photo by Fotosearch.com
Page iii	Photo by Dreamstime.com
Page v	Photo by istockphoto.com
Page 1	Photo by istockphoto.com
Page 2	Photo by Dreamstime.com
Page 3	Photo by istockphoto.com
Page 4	Photo by Dreamstime.com
Page 5	Photo by istockphoto.com
Page 6	Photo by Vergie Hughes
Page 7	Photo by Dreamstime.com
Page 8	Photo by Tosha Francis of The Captured Life Photography
Page 9	Photo by Dreamstime.com
Page 10	Photo used with permission by Medela, Inc.
Page 14	Photo by Dreamstime.com
Page 16	Photo by Dreamstime.com
Page 17	Photo by Dreamstime.com
Page 19	Photo by Lucille Weinstat
Page 20	Photo by Dreamstime.com
Page 21	Photo by Dreamstime.com
Page 25	Photo by istockphoto.com
Page 26	Photo by istockphoto.com
Page 29	Photo by Michael J. N. Bowles
Page 30	Photo by Dreamstime.com
Page 31	Photo used with permission by Medela, Inc.
Back Cover	Photo by Fotosearch.com

For More Information

Books

Bolster, Alice. *Fatherwise: 101 Tips for a New Father.* Schaumburg, IL: La Leche League International, 2000.

Buescher, E. Stephen, MD. *Breastfeeding and Diseases: A Reference Guide.* Amarillo, Texas: Hale Publishing, L.P., 2008.

Brott, Armin A. *The New Father: A Dad's Guide to the First Year.* New York: Abbeville Press, 1997.

di Properzio, James, Jennifer Margulis, and Christopher Briscoe. *The Baby Bonding Book for Dads : Building a Closer Connection with Your Baby.* New York: Willow Creek Press, Inc., 2008.

Glennon, Will. *Fathering: Strengthening Connection with Your Children No Matter Where You Are.* York Beach, ME: Conari Press, 1995.

Goldman, Marcus Jacob, MD. *The Joy of Fatherhood: The First Twelve Months.* New York: Prima Publishing, 2000.

Hale, Thomas W., PhD. *A Medication Guide for Breastfeeding Moms.* Amarillo, TX: Pharmasoft Medical Publishing, 2005.

Hale, Thomas W., PhD. *Medications and Mothers' Milk: A Manual of Lactational Pharmacology.* Amarillo, TX: Pharmasoft Medical Publishing, 2008.

Heinowitz, Jack. *Pregnant Fathers: Becoming the Father You Want to Be.* Kansas City, MO: Andrews McMeel Publishing, 1997.

Levine, Suzanne Braun. *Father's Courage: What Happens When Men Put Family First.* Harcourt, 2000.

McKenna, James J., *Sleeping With Your Baby: A Parent's Guide to Cosleeping,* Platypus Media, Washington, DC 2006.

Mohrbacher, Nancy, and Julie Stock. *The Breastfeeding Answer Book.* Ed. Judy Torgus. New York: La Leche League International, 1997.

Pruett, Kyle D. *Fatherneed: Why Father Care Is As Essential As Mother Care for Your Child.* New York: Broadway Books, 2001.

Sears, Robert, James M. Sears, and William Sears. *Father's First Steps : 25 Things Every New Dad Should Know.* New York: Harvard Common P, 2006.

Sears, William, MD. *Keys to Becoming a Father.* Hauppauge, NY: Barrons, 1991.

West, Diana, and Lisa Marasco. *The Breastfeeding Mother's Guide to Making More Milk.* New York: McGraw-Hill Companies, 2008

West, Diana, and Subbadra Tidball. *Defining Your Own Success : Breastfeeding after Breast Reduction Surgery.* New York: La Leche League International, 2001.

For More Information *continued*

Videos

Breastfeeding and Basketball, InJoy Videos, Boulder, CO, 1999. http://injoyvideos.com/product.php?proid=89&page=Breastfeeding_& _Basketball

Fathers Supporting Breastfeeding: A Video in Support of African American Breastfeeding, USDA Food and Nutrition Service. Available at no cost as long as supplies last. www.fns.usda.gov/wic/Fathers/ SupportingBreastfeeding.HTM

Fathers Matter, Noodle Soup, Cleveland, Ohio, 1998. Available at http://www.noodlesoup.com/fathersmattervideo.aspx.

The Dad Difference, InJoy Videos, Boulder, CO, 2004. Available at http://www.injoyvideos.com/product.php?proid=32&sub_catid=6&page=The_Dad_Difference

Organizations and Websites

Ameda (www.ameda.com) offers many tools that lead to a fulfilling breastfeeding experience – articles that give you the ins and outs of breastfeeding and breast pumping, along with a community of other parents who can share their stories.

American Academy of Pediatrics (www.aap.org) is made up of 60,000 pediatricians committed to the attainment of optimal physical, mental, and social health and well-being for all infants, children, adolescents, and young adults.

Australian Breastfeeding Association – Just for Fathers (www.breastfeeding.asn.au/bfinfo/father.html) is an organization of breastfeeding women and their partners, along with health professionals – all interested in the protection and promotion of breastfeeding.

Boot Camp for New Dads (http://www.bootcampfornewdads.org/) is a unique father-to-father, community-based workshop that inspires and equips men of different economic levels, ages, and cultures to become confidently engaged with their infants, support their peers, and personally navigate their transformation into dads.

Drugs and Lactation Database (LactMed) (http://toxnet.nlm.nih.gov/cgi-bin/sis/htmlgen?LACT) by the U.S. National Library of Medicine is a peer-reviewed and fully referenced database of drugs to which breastfeeding mothers may be exposed. Among the data included are maternal and infant levels of drugs, possible effects on breastfed infants and on lactation, and alternate drugs to consider.

Fathers and Families Coalition of America, Inc. (www.azffc.org) is a premiere national one-stop resource for those who seek to improve the outcomes for children through healthy fathers and family interaction.

Fathers Supporting Breastfeeding (www.fns.usda.gov/wic/Fathers/SupportingBreastfeeding.HTM) is a Food and Nutrition Service project targeted to African American fathers so that they may positively impact a mother's decision to breastfeed.

La Leche League (www.llli.org) has a rich history and an established philosophy of mothering through breastfeeding. Also see **La Leche League – Fathers and Breastfeeding** (www.llli.org/NB/NBfathers.html) for articles on the father's role in the breastfeeding relationship.

Medela Breastfeeding (www.medelabreastfeedingus.com/) continues to lead the industry through the development of innovative and high-quality breastfeeding and phototherapy products, human lactation research, and education.

National Fatherhood Initiative (www.fatherhood.org) strives to improve the well being of children by increasing the promotion of children growing up with involved, responsible, and committed fathers.

U.S. Department of Health – Healthy People 2010 (www.healthypeople.gov) is a set of health objectives for the Nation to achieve over the first decade of the new century, challenging everyone to take specific steps to ensure that good health, as well as long life, are enjoyed by all.

World Alliance for Breastfeeding Action: Men's Initiative (www.waba.org.my/whatwedo/mensinitiative/) hopes to create an enabling environment where men, particularly fathers, participate actively and share responsibilities with women in optimally caring for their infants and young children, through advocacy, education and capacity building.

About the Executive Editor

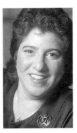

An award-winning science and parenting writer, Dia L. Michels is the co-author of *Breastfeeding At A Glance: Facts, Figures and Trivia about Breastfeeding*, and *Milk, Money & Madness: The Culture and Politics of Breastfeeding*. She is author of *If My Mom Were a Platypus: Mammal Babies and Their Mothers*, *101 Things Everyone Should Know About Science* and the 5-book *Look What I See! Where Can I Be?* series for young children (which include images of breastfeeding, baby-wearing, family beds and active fathering). A popular speaker, Dia has delivered speeches at national and international healthcare and parenting conferences. She also teaches classes at children's, natural history, and science museums around the U.S. Dia lives in Washington, DC with her husband and their three children. She can be reached at Dia@PlatypusMedia.com.

Special Thanks to the Contributing Editors

Platypus Media would like to extend a heartfelt thanks to our Contributing Editors, who worked so diligently to ensure that the information presented is both accurate and interesting.

Stine Bauer Dahlberg, Sjotorp, Sweden

Katy Lebbing, BS, IBCLC, RLC, Villa Park, IL, USA

Judy Torgus, LLL Leader, River Grove, IL, USA

Tracey Kilby, Washington, DC

Additional Parenting Guides
Available From Platypus Media

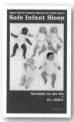

Coming soon! *What Every Parent Needs to Know about Safe Infant Sleep*

Infant safety during waking hours is well documented and information is readily available; however, infant safety during sleeping hours is another matter entirely. Experts give mixed messages on if, and when, a baby should sleep in the same bed as his parents, the same room as his parents, or in a crib in a separate room. *What Every Parent Needs to Know about Safe Infant Sleep* educates parents on the pros and cons of different sleep.

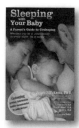

Sleeping with Your Baby: A Parent's Guide to Cosleeping, **James J. McKenna, PhD**

Walking readers through various ways to safely cosleep, whether bedsharing or not, *Sleeping with Your Baby* provides the latest information on the potential scientific benefits of cosleeping. Complete with sections on minimizing hazards and risks, world-wide recognized cosleeping authority, James J. McKenna, explains why and how to sleep with your baby.

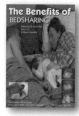

The Benefits of Bedsharing DVD, by
Dr. Helen Ball, Sally Inch and Marion Copeland

This DVD explains that if done safely, bedsharing allows mothers to respond in seconds, instead of minutes, to their baby's needs. Most breastfeeding mothers around the world sleep with their babies, yet modern beds are designed for adult comfort, not infant safety. *The Benefits of Bedsharing* features a variety of mothers and fathers cosleeping at home, as well as in hospital environments, to reinforce the importance and the benefits of safe bedsharing.

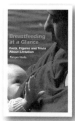

Breastfeeding at a Glance: Facts, Figures and Trivia about Lactation, by **Dia L. Michels and Cynthia Good Mojab, MS, with Naomi Bromberg Bar-Yam, PhD**

This handy booklet answers frequently asked questions about breastfeeding; lists benefits for mother, baby and community; and provides information on mammal lactation, breastfeeding and the law, a resource list, breastfeeding rates and more.

About Platypus Media

Platypus Media is an independent publisher dedicated to promoting family life by creating and distributing high quality materials about families. We strive to be the premier source of products that have a broad appeal to families and the professionals who work with them. We celebrate the importance of family closeness to the full and healthy development of children. Our goal is to bring materials to the market that parents love, children enjoy, teachers appreciate, and parenting professionals value. Platypus Media currently offers a selection of books, booklets, videos, DVDs and other products, many of which have garnered widespread praise. For more information about our publications, bulk purchasing, or to request a catalog, visit us at www.PlatypusMedia.com.

Platypus Media is committed to the promotion and protection of breastfeeding. We donate six percent of our profits to breastfeeding organizations.

Platypus Media
725 8th Street SE
Washington, DC 20003
Toll-free: 1-877-PLATYPS (1-877-752-8977)
Tel: 202-546-1674
Fax: 202-546-2356
www.PlatypusMedia.com
Info@PlatypusMedia.com

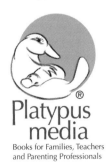

Platypus
media
Books for Families, Teachers
and Parenting Professionals